Free Book Offer:

Get How to be a Super Mom For Free

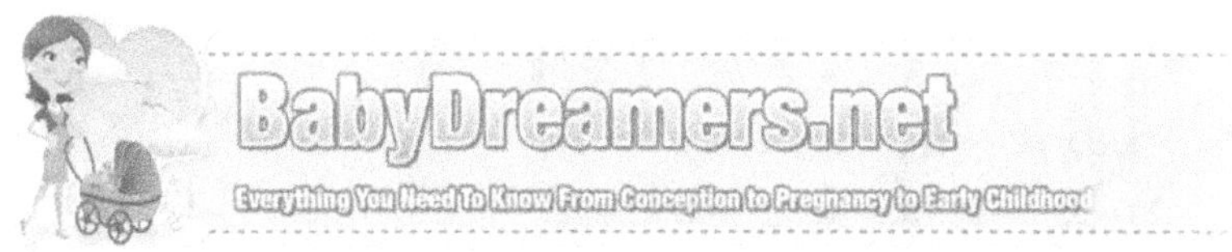

A Short Read is a type of book that is designed to be read in one quick sitting.

These no fluff books are perfect for people who want an overview about a subject in a short period of time.

Table of Contents

The Emotional Rollercoaster of Trying to Conceive

The journey of trying to conceive a baby can be an emotional rollercoaster for couples. It is a time filled with hope, excitement, and anticipation, but also with disappointment, anxiety, and stress. The ups and downs of this journey can take a toll on the emotional well-being of both partners, as they navigate through the complexities of fertility challenges.

One of the most challenging aspects of trying to conceive is dealing with disappointment. Each negative pregnancy test or failed fertility treatment can be a devastating blow, leaving couples feeling discouraged and disheartened. It is important to acknowledge and process these emotions, allowing space for grief and sadness, while also finding ways to stay hopeful and optimistic.

Managing anxiety and stress is another crucial aspect of the emotional journey of trying to conceive. The pressure to conceive can be overwhelming, both from societal expectations and personal desires. Couples may feel the weight of this pressure and experience heightened levels of anxiety and stress. It is essential to find healthy coping mechanisms to navigate through these emotions, such as engaging in relaxation techniques, pursuing hobbies and interests, and seeking support from loved ones or professional counseling.

The emotional rollercoaster of trying to conceive can also be intensified by the expectations of family, friends, and society. Coping with these expectations can be challenging, as couples may feel the need to constantly update others on their progress or face judgment and scrutiny. It is important to establish boundaries and communicate openly with loved ones about the emotional journey, seeking their understanding and support.

Furthermore, the process of trying to conceive can sometimes lead to feelings of self-blame and guilt. Couples may question themselves and wonder if they are doing something wrong or if there is something inherently wrong with them. It is crucial to address these feelings and remind oneself that infertility is a complex issue that is not solely the individual's fault. Seeking professional guidance and support can be helpful in navigating through these emotions and finding ways to cope.

Throughout this emotional journey, it is essential for couples to support and comfort each other. They can provide a safe space for each other to express their emotions and be there to offer comfort and understanding. By leaning on one another, couples can find strength and resilience in the face of challenges and setbacks.

Despite the emotional challenges, it is important to hold onto hope and optimism. Celebrating small victories along the way, even if pregnancy has not yet been achieved, can help maintain a positive mindset. Additionally, exploring alternative paths to parenthood, such as adoption or assisted reproductive technologies, can provide a sense of empowerment and open new possibilities.

Dealing with grief and loss is also a part of the emotional journey of trying to conceive. Miscarriage and infertility can bring about intense emotions of grief and heartbreak. It is important to process these emotions and find ways to heal and move forward. Seeking support from others who have experienced similar losses can be invaluable in this process.

Overall, the emotional rollercoaster of trying to conceive is a complex and challenging journey. It requires couples to navigate through a range of emotions, from hope and excitement to disappointment and grief. By finding healthy coping mechanisms, seeking support, and nurturing open communication, couples can navigate this emotional rollercoaster together and find ways to support each other along the way.

Dealing with Disappointment

Dealing with disappointment can be one of the most challenging aspects of the journey to conceive. Each negative pregnancy test or failed fertility treatment can bring a wave of complex emotions that can be overwhelming. It is important to navigate these emotions in a healthy and supportive way.

One way to cope with disappointment is to allow yourself to feel the emotions fully. It is natural to feel sadness, frustration, and even anger when faced with setbacks on the path to conception. Acknowledging and accepting these emotions can be a crucial step in the healing process.

It can also be helpful to seek support from your partner, friends, or a support group. Talking about your feelings and experiences with others who are going through a similar journey can provide comfort and understanding. Sharing your struggles and receiving empathy can help alleviate some of the emotional burden.

Additionally, finding healthy coping mechanisms can make a significant difference in managing disappointment. Engaging in self-care activities such as exercise, meditation, or pursuing hobbies can help reduce stress and promote emotional well-being. It is important to prioritize your own needs and take time for yourself.

Remember, dealing with disappointment is a normal part of the process. It is essential to be patient and kind to yourself as you navigate the ups and downs of trying to conceive. With the right support and coping strategies, you can find the strength to continue on your journey towards parenthood.

Managing Anxiety and Stress

Trying to conceive can be an emotional rollercoaster, and one of the biggest challenges couples face is managing anxiety and stress. The journey to parenthood can be filled with uncertainty, disappointment, and frustration, which can take a toll on one's mental and emotional well-being. It's important to find healthy coping mechanisms to navigate these emotions and reduce anxiety and stress.

One effective way to manage anxiety and stress is to prioritize self-care. Taking care of your physical and mental health can have a positive impact on your overall well-being. Engaging in relaxation techniques such as meditation, yoga, or deep breathing exercises can help reduce stress levels and promote emotional well-being. These practices can help you find a sense of calm and provide a much-needed break from the pressures of trying to conceive.

Another helpful strategy is to pursue hobbies and interests outside of the realm of trying to conceive. Engaging in activities that bring you joy and fulfillment can provide a much-needed distraction from the stress and anxiety of the journey. Whether it's painting, gardening, or playing a musical instrument, finding time for activities that bring you happiness can help shift your focus and improve your emotional well-being.

It's also important to communicate openly with your partner about your emotions and feelings. Expressing your worries, fears, and frustrations can help foster understanding and support between you and your partner. It's natural for partners to have different ways of coping with the emotional rollercoaster, so finding common ground and supporting each other's coping mechanisms is crucial.

Additionally, seeking professional counseling and therapy can be beneficial for managing anxiety and stress. A trained therapist can provide guidance, support, and strategies for coping with the emotional challenges of trying to conceive. They can help you navigate the ups and downs of the journey and provide a safe space to express your emotions.

Remember, managing anxiety and stress is essential for your overall well-being during the process of trying to conceive. Finding healthy coping mechanisms, prioritizing self-care, and seeking support can make a significant difference in your emotional journey. Take care of yourself, be patient, and remember that you're not alone in this journey.

The Pressure to Conceive

The journey to conceive a baby can be filled with immense pressure, both from society and within oneself. Couples often face societal expectations and personal desires to start a family, which can create a significant emotional toll. The pressure to conceive can come from various sources, including well-meaning family members, friends, and even strangers who inquire about plans for children. This constant external pressure can lead to feelings of inadequacy, guilt, and self-doubt.

Additionally, couples may put pressure on themselves to conceive, feeling a deep desire to experience the joy of parenthood. They may feel a sense of urgency as they see friends and acquaintances starting families, which can intensify the emotional strain. The fear of missing out on the opportunity to have a child can create a sense of desperation and anxiety.

It is important to recognize the impact that the pressure to conceive can have on emotional well-being. The constant focus on fertility and the inability to conceive can lead to heightened stress levels, feelings of failure, and a sense of loss. Couples may find themselves constantly analyzing every aspect of their lives, from their diet and exercise routines to their intimacy and timing of intercourse, in an effort to increase their chances of conception.

It is crucial for couples to navigate these pressures and prioritize their emotional well-being throughout the journey of trying to conceive. This may involve setting boundaries with others, seeking support from loved ones or professionals, and finding healthy coping mechanisms to manage stress and anxiety. It is important to remember that each individual and couple's journey is unique, and there is no one-size-fits-all approach to conceiving a baby.

Coping with Expectations

When trying to conceive, couples often find themselves facing a barrage of expectations from family, friends, and society. These expectations can add an additional layer of pressure and stress to an already emotionally challenging journey. Coping with these expectations is crucial for maintaining one's emotional well-being and preserving the bond between partners.

One strategy for managing expectations is setting boundaries. It's important to communicate openly with loved ones about your journey and let them know what level of involvement or support you are comfortable with. This can help prevent unwanted advice or intrusive questions that may contribute to feelings of frustration or inadequacy.

Another helpful approach is to focus on your own goals and desires. Remember that this journey is about you and your partner, and it's important to prioritize your own well-being and happiness above societal expectations. This may involve taking a step back from social events or gatherings that may trigger negative emotions or comparisons.

Creating a support network of individuals who understand and empathize with your situation can also be beneficial. Joining an infertility support group or seeking therapy can provide a safe space to share your experiences, gain perspective, and receive guidance from others who are going through similar challenges.

Lastly, practicing self-compassion is key. It's important to remind yourself that you are doing the best you can and that your worth is not defined by your ability to conceive. Be gentle with yourself and allow yourself to feel a range of emotions without judgment.

By implementing these strategies, couples can navigate the expectations of family, friends, and society while trying to conceive, ultimately preserving their emotional well-being and strengthening their relationship.

Dealing with Self-Blame

Addressing the feelings of guilt and self-blame that can arise when struggling to conceive can be a challenging and emotional journey. It is common for individuals and couples experiencing difficulties in conceiving to question themselves and wonder if they are somehow to blame for their struggles. These feelings can be overwhelming and can have a significant impact on one's emotional well-being.

It is important to remember that infertility is a complex medical condition that can have various causes, many of which are beyond an individual's control. Blaming oneself for not being able to conceive is not productive or fair. Instead, it is crucial to shift the focus towards understanding and compassion.

One way to address self-blame is by seeking support from loved ones, professionals, or support groups who can provide reassurance and understanding. Talking openly about one's feelings and experiences can help alleviate the burden of guilt and self-blame. Sharing with others who have gone through similar struggles can provide a sense of validation and remind individuals that they are not alone in their journey.

Additionally, practicing self-compassion is essential. It is important to remind oneself that struggling to conceive does not define one's worth as a person or partner. Taking time for self-care, engaging in activities that bring joy and fulfillment, and nurturing emotional well-being can help combat feelings of self-blame.

Furthermore, seeking professional help from therapists or counselors who specialize in infertility can be beneficial. They can provide guidance and support in navigating the complex emotions associated with self-blame and help develop coping strategies to manage these feelings effectively.

Remember, struggling to conceive is not a reflection of personal failure. It is a challenging journey that requires strength, resilience, and support. By addressing self-blame and embracing self-compassion, individuals and couples can find healing and move forward on their path to parenthood.

Supporting Each Other

When embarking on the emotional journey of trying to conceive, it is crucial for couples to come together and provide support and comfort to one another. This rollercoaster of emotions can be overwhelming, but by standing united, couples can navigate the ups and downs with strength and resilience.

One way couples can support each other is by creating a safe space for open and honest communication. This means actively listening to each other's fears, frustrations, and hopes without judgment. By validating each other's emotions and experiences, couples can build a strong foundation of trust and understanding.

Additionally, finding shared coping mechanisms can be incredibly beneficial. Whether it's going for walks together, practicing relaxation techniques, or engaging in a hobby as a couple, finding activities that bring comfort and joy can help alleviate stress and strengthen the bond between partners.

It's also important for couples to acknowledge and respect each other's individual needs during this journey. Each person may have different ways of processing emotions and dealing with stress. By recognizing and supporting these differences, couples can ensure that both partners feel heard and valued.

Furthermore, seeking outside support can be immensely helpful. Joining a support group for couples trying to conceive or seeking professional therapy can provide a safe space to share experiences, gain insights, and learn coping strategies. These resources can offer guidance and encouragement, reminding couples that they are not alone in their journey.

Finally, celebrating small victories together can be a powerful way to support each other. Whether it's a positive fertility test result, reaching a milestone in the fertility treatment process, or simply finding moments of joy and connection amidst the challenges, acknowledging and celebrating these moments can provide a much-needed boost of hope and optimism.

Supporting each other throughout the emotional journey of trying to conceive is crucial for maintaining a strong and resilient partnership. By creating a foundation of open communication, shared coping mechanisms, and seeking outside support, couples can navigate the highs and lows together, finding strength in each other's love and support.

Hope and Optimism

When faced with challenges and setbacks on the path to conception, maintaining hope and optimism can be a powerful tool for couples. It is important to remember that the journey to parenthood is not always a linear one, and there may be obstacles along the way. However, by cultivating hope and optimism, couples can navigate these challenges with resilience and determination.

One way to find hope and optimism is by celebrating the small victories. Even if pregnancy has not yet been achieved, it is important to recognize and appreciate the milestones and achievements along the way. This could include reaching a certain point in the fertility treatment process, receiving positive feedback from doctors, or simply taking proactive steps towards conception. By acknowledging these small victories, couples can stay motivated and hopeful, knowing that progress is being made.

Another way to maintain hope and optimism is by exploring alternative paths to parenthood. Sometimes, conception proves to be difficult despite the best efforts. In such cases, considering options like adoption or assisted reproductive technologies can provide a renewed sense of hope. These alternative paths may offer different challenges and setbacks, but they also open up new possibilities for starting a family. By embracing these alternatives, couples can find hope in the idea that their dream of parenthood can still come true, albeit in a different way.

Lastly, it is important to remember that hope and optimism are not static. They require active cultivation and nourishment. This can be done through self-care and emotional well-being practices. Engaging in relaxation techniques such as meditation, yoga, or deep breathing can help reduce stress and promote a positive mindset. Pursuing hobbies and interests outside of the realm of trying to conceive can also bring joy and fulfillment, reminding couples that their happiness is not solely dependent on becoming parents.

In conclusion, finding and maintaining hope and optimism on the path to conception is crucial for couples. By celebrating small victories, exploring alternative paths, and prioritizing self-care, couples can stay resilient and positive in the face of challenges and setbacks. Remember, hope is not lost as long as optimism is alive.

Celebrating Small Victories

Celebrating small victories is an important part of the emotional journey of trying to conceive. While the ultimate goal may be to achieve pregnancy, it's essential to recognize and appreciate the small milestones and achievements along the way, even if pregnancy has not yet been achieved.

These small victories can take many forms. It could be a month of consistently tracking ovulation and having a regular menstrual cycle. It could be receiving a positive result from an ovulation predictor kit or having a successful fertility treatment cycle. It could be reaching out for support and joining an infertility support group. Each of these milestones is a step forward in the journey, and they deserve to be celebrated.

One way to celebrate small victories is to create a list of accomplishments. This can be done individually or as a couple. Write down each milestone or achievement, no matter how small it may seem. Seeing these accomplishments on paper can help provide a sense of progress and motivation to keep going.

Another way to celebrate is to treat yourself. Take time to do something that brings you joy and relaxation. It could be a spa day, a weekend getaway, or simply indulging in your favorite dessert. By taking care of yourself and acknowledging your efforts, you are reinforcing the importance of self-care and emotional well-being throughout the journey.

Additionally, it's important to share these small victories with your partner, family, and friends. They can offer support, encouragement, and celebrate with you. Having a support system that understands the challenges and milestones can make the journey feel less lonely and overwhelming.

Remember, celebrating small victories is not about minimizing the challenges or frustrations that come with trying to conceive. It's about finding moments of joy and progress amidst the ups and downs. By recognizing and appreciating these small milestones, you are nurturing hope, resilience, and emotional well-being on the path to conception.

Exploring Alternative Paths

When conception proves difficult, it can be a challenging and emotional journey for couples. However, it's important to remember that there are alternative paths to parenthood that can be explored and embraced. One option is adoption, which allows couples to provide a loving home for a child in need. Adoption can be a beautiful and fulfilling way to become parents, offering the opportunity to create a family and make a positive impact on a child's life.

Another alternative path is assisted reproductive technologies, which can help couples overcome fertility challenges. These technologies include procedures such as in vitro fertilization (IVF), where eggs and sperm are combined in a laboratory and then transferred to the uterus. Other options include intrauterine insemination (IUI) and surrogacy. Assisted reproductive technologies have helped many couples achieve their dream of parenthood, offering hope and possibilities when natural conception is not possible.

Exploring alternative paths to parenthood requires careful consideration and research. It's important to gather information, consult with medical professionals, and seek support from others who have gone through similar experiences. Each couple's journey is unique, and what works for one may not work for another. By considering and embracing alternative paths, couples can find new avenues to fulfill their desire to become parents and create a loving family.

Dealing with Grief and Loss

Dealing with Grief and Loss

Navigating the complex emotions of grief and loss can be incredibly challenging for couples facing miscarriage or infertility. These experiences can evoke a range of intense emotions, including sadness, anger, guilt, and even feelings of emptiness. It is important for individuals and couples to acknowledge and process these emotions in a healthy and supportive way.

When faced with a miscarriage, the loss of a pregnancy can be devastating. It is a deeply personal and emotional experience that can leave individuals feeling overwhelmed and heartbroken. It is important to remember that grief is a natural response to loss, and it is okay to allow yourself to grieve and mourn the loss of the pregnancy.

Infertility, on the other hand, can bring about its own unique set of emotions. The inability to conceive can lead to feelings of inadequacy, frustration, and a sense of loss. It is important for individuals and couples to recognize that these feelings are valid and to seek support from loved ones or professional resources.

During this difficult time, it can be helpful to engage in self-care activities that promote emotional healing and well-being. This may include seeking therapy or counseling, joining support groups, or finding solace in creative outlets such as writing or art. It is also important to communicate openly with your partner about your emotions and to support each other through the grieving process.

Remember, grief and loss are deeply personal experiences, and there is no right or wrong way to navigate them. Each individual and couple will have their own unique journey, and it is important to be patient and kind to yourself as you work through these emotions. With time, support, and self-care, it is possible to find healing and move forward on your path to parenthood or alternative paths to fulfillment.

Processing Miscarriage

Processing Miscarriage

Coping with the emotional aftermath of a miscarriage can be incredibly challenging. Miscarriage is a devastating loss, and it is important to allow yourself to grieve and process the emotions that arise. It is normal to feel a wide range of emotions such as sadness, anger, guilt, and even numbness. Each person's experience is unique, and it is essential to give yourself the time and space to heal.

One way to cope with the emotional aftermath of a miscarriage is to seek support from loved ones or join a support group specifically for individuals who have experienced pregnancy loss. Talking with others who have gone through a similar experience can provide comfort and understanding. Additionally, professional counseling or therapy can be beneficial in navigating the complex emotions associated with miscarriage.

It is also important to take care of yourself physically during this time. Engaging in self-care activities such as exercise, getting enough rest, and eating a healthy diet can help support your overall well-being. It is crucial to be patient with yourself and allow yourself to heal at your own pace.

Remember that healing is a process, and it is okay to have good days and bad days. Be gentle with yourself and give yourself permission to feel and process your emotions. Over time, the pain may lessen, and you may find ways to honor the memory of your lost pregnancy while finding hope for the future.

Coming to Terms with Infertility

Coming to terms with infertility can be an incredibly challenging and emotional journey. When faced with a diagnosis of infertility, couples may experience a wide range of emotions, including sadness, anger, frustration, and even a sense of loss. It is important for individuals and couples to give themselves permission to grieve and process these emotions.

Acceptance is a key step in coming to terms with infertility. It involves acknowledging the reality of the situation and understanding that conceiving a biological child may not be possible. This can be a difficult realization to come to, but it is an important part of the healing process.

Exploring options for moving forward is another crucial aspect of coming to terms with infertility. There are a variety of alternative paths to parenthood that individuals and couples can consider, such as adoption or assisted reproductive technologies like in vitro fertilization (IVF). It can be helpful to research and gather information about these options, seeking guidance from medical professionals and fertility specialists.

Additionally, seeking emotional support is essential during this time. Joining an infertility support group or seeking individual therapy can provide a safe space to share experiences, emotions, and coping strategies with others who are going through similar challenges. Talking openly with loved ones about the emotional journey of infertility can also be beneficial, as it can foster understanding and support.

It is important to remember that coming to terms with infertility is a deeply personal process, and everyone's journey will be unique. There is no right or wrong way to navigate this emotional rollercoaster, and it is okay to take the time needed to heal and find peace with the situation. By accepting and processing the emotions that arise, exploring alternative paths to parenthood, and seeking support, individuals and couples can find a way forward and create a fulfilling life beyond infertility.

Seeking Support

When facing the emotional challenges of trying to conceive, seeking support is crucial. Finding and utilizing support networks can provide a much-needed source of comfort, understanding, and guidance throughout the journey. One valuable resource is infertility support groups, where individuals and couples going through similar experiences can come together to share their stories, offer advice, and provide emotional support.

Infertility support groups create a safe space for individuals to express their feelings, fears, and frustrations without judgment. It can be incredibly empowering to connect with others who truly understand the ups and downs of the fertility journey. These groups often meet in person or online, allowing for flexibility and accessibility for individuals in different locations.

Therapy is another valuable form of support for couples trying to conceive. Working with a therapist who specializes in infertility can provide a confidential space to explore and process the complex emotions that arise during this time. A therapist can offer guidance, coping strategies, and tools to help individuals and couples navigate the emotional rollercoaster of trying to conceive.

Additionally, seeking support from loved ones is essential. Communicating openly with family and friends about the emotional challenges of trying to conceive can foster understanding and empathy. Loved ones can provide a listening ear, offer words of encouragement, and be a source of comfort during difficult times.

In conclusion, finding and utilizing support networks, such as infertility support groups or therapy, can be instrumental in navigating the emotional challenges of trying to conceive. These resources provide a sense of community, understanding, and guidance, helping individuals and couples feel less alone in their journey towards parenthood.

Opening Up to Loved Ones

Opening up to loved ones about the emotional journey of trying to conceive is an important step in seeking understanding and support. It can be difficult to share such personal and vulnerable experiences, but having a strong support system can make a significant difference in navigating the ups and downs of the process.

When communicating with family and friends, it's important to approach the conversation with honesty and vulnerability. Let them know how you are feeling and what you are going through, allowing them to understand the emotional toll that trying to conceive can have. This can help bridge the gap between your experiences and their understanding, fostering empathy and support.

Creating a safe space for open dialogue is crucial. Encourage your loved ones to ask questions and express their own feelings, allowing for a two-way conversation. This can help them better understand your perspective and provide the support that you need.

It's important to remember that not everyone will fully understand or know how to respond. Some may unintentionally say things that are hurtful or dismissive. In these situations, try to approach the conversation with patience and educate them about your experience. Providing resources or directing them to support groups or educational materials can help them gain a better understanding.

Seeking support from loved ones can also extend beyond just emotional support. They may be able to offer practical help, such as accompanying you to doctor's appointments or helping with household tasks. Don't hesitate to communicate your needs and let them know how they can best support you.

Ultimately, opening up to loved ones about the emotional journey of trying to conceive can help strengthen your support system and provide a sense of comfort and understanding. Remember, you don't have to face this journey alone.

Professional Counseling and Therapy

Professional counseling and therapy can play a crucial role in managing the emotional toll of trying to conceive. It provides a safe and supportive space for individuals and couples to explore their feelings, fears, and frustrations related to the journey of trying to conceive.

One of the benefits of professional counseling and therapy is that it offers a non-judgmental environment where individuals can express their emotions freely. The therapist or counselor can help individuals navigate through the complex emotions that arise during this challenging time, such as grief, anxiety, and depression.

During counseling sessions, individuals can gain a better understanding of their emotions and develop coping strategies to deal with the ups and downs of trying to conceive. Therapists can provide guidance on stress management techniques, communication skills, and self-care practices that can help individuals maintain their emotional well-being.

Additionally, counseling and therapy can also help individuals and couples strengthen their relationship. The process of trying to conceive can put a strain on even the strongest partnerships, but therapy sessions can provide a space for open and honest communication. Couples can learn how to support each other, manage differences in coping mechanisms, and navigate the challenges together.

It's important to remember that seeking professional help is not a sign of weakness, but rather a proactive step towards taking care of one's emotional well-being. Just as individuals seek medical assistance for physical health issues, seeking counseling or therapy for emotional support is equally important.

In conclusion, professional counseling and therapy can be a valuable resource for individuals and couples who are trying to conceive. It offers a supportive environment to explore emotions, develop coping strategies, and strengthen relationships. By seeking professional help, individuals can better manage the emotional toll of trying to conceive and find support in their journey towards parenthood.

Dealing with Jealousy and Resentment

Dealing with jealousy and resentment can be one of the most challenging aspects of the emotional rollercoaster of trying to conceive. It is natural to feel a mix of emotions when others around you achieve pregnancy or parenthood while you are still on your own journey. These complex emotions can range from envy and bitterness to sadness and frustration.

One way to address these feelings is by acknowledging and accepting them. It is okay to feel jealous or resentful, as long as you don't let these emotions consume you. Recognize that it is normal to have these emotions, but also remind yourself that everyone's journey is different and comparing yourself to others will only bring more negativity.

It can also be helpful to shift your perspective and focus on your own journey. Instead of dwelling on what others have, try to appreciate the unique aspects of your own life. Celebrate your own accomplishments and milestones, no matter how small they may seem. Remember that your worth and happiness are not defined by whether or not you are able to conceive.

- Practice gratitude: Take time each day to reflect on the things you are grateful for in your life. This can help shift your focus away from jealousy and resentment.
- Seek support: Reach out to others who are going through a similar experience. Joining a support group or connecting with others online can provide a safe space to share your feelings and gain perspective.
- Practice self-care: Take care of yourself both physically and emotionally. Engage in activities that bring you joy and help you relax. This can

help alleviate feelings of jealousy and resentment.

Remember, it is important to be kind to yourself during this emotional journey. Allow yourself to feel and process these complex emotions, but also remember to focus on your own well-being and happiness.

Managing Social Media Triggers

Managing Social Media Triggers

Social media has become an integral part of our lives, allowing us to connect with others, share our experiences, and stay updated on the latest trends. However, for couples trying to conceive, social media can also be a source of jealousy and resentment. Seeing pregnancy announcements, baby photos, and parenting milestones can trigger a range of emotions, from sadness and frustration to envy and self-doubt.

It's important for couples to develop strategies to navigate social media in a way that protects their emotional well-being. Here are some tips to help manage social media triggers:

- Limit Your Exposure: Consider taking breaks from social media or unfollowing accounts that frequently post pregnancy or parenting content. This can help create a healthier online environment for you.

- Focus on Your Journey: Remember that everyone's path to parenthood is unique. Instead of comparing yourself to others, focus on your own journey and the progress you are making.
- Seek Support: Connect with others who are going through a similar experience by joining online support groups or forums. Surrounding yourself with understanding and supportive individuals can help alleviate feelings of isolation and provide a safe space to share your emotions.
- Practice Self-Care: Engage in activities that bring you joy and help you relax. This could include hobbies, exercise, spending time in nature, or practicing mindfulness techniques such as meditation or deep breathing.

Remember, social media is a curated space where people often highlight the positive aspects of their lives. It's important to take everything you see with a grain of salt and remember that real life is often more complex and nuanced than what is portrayed online. By being mindful of your social media usage and implementing strategies to manage triggers, you can protect your emotional well-being and focus on your own journey towards conception.

Shifting Perspective

When trying to conceive, it's easy to get caught up in the rollercoaster of emotions and become consumed by the desire for a baby. However, shifting perspective can be a powerful tool in maintaining emotional well-being throughout this journey. Instead of solely focusing on the end goal of pregnancy, it's important to also prioritize personal growth and happiness.

One way to shift perspective is to remind yourself of the things that bring you joy and fulfillment outside of trying to conceive. Engaging in hobbies and interests that you love can provide a much-needed distraction and help you find a sense of purpose beyond parenthood. Whether it's painting, hiking, or playing a musical instrument, these activities can bring a sense of fulfillment and happiness, reminding you that there is more to life than just trying to conceive.

Another way to shift perspective is to practice gratitude and focus on the positive aspects of your life. Take time each day to reflect on the things you are grateful for, whether it's the support of your partner, the love of your family and friends, or the beauty of nature. By shifting your focus to the blessings in your life, you can cultivate a sense of gratitude and contentment, even in the midst of the challenges of trying to conceive.

It's also important to remember that personal growth and happiness are ongoing journeys. Take time to invest in yourself and prioritize self-care. This may involve engaging in relaxation techniques such as meditation or yoga, which can help reduce stress and promote emotional well-being. Additionally, seeking support from a therapist or counselor can provide a safe space to explore your emotions and develop coping strategies.

By shifting perspective and focusing on personal growth and happiness, you can navigate the emotional rollercoaster of trying to conceive with a greater sense of balance and fulfillment. Remember, the journey to parenthood is not just about the end result, but also about the growth and self-discovery along the way.

Self-Care and Emotional Well-being

During the emotional rollercoaster of trying to conceive, it is crucial to prioritize self-care and emotional well-being. This journey can be filled with ups and downs, and taking care of yourself is essential for maintaining your overall health and happiness. Here are some strategies to help you prioritize self-care and emotional well-being throughout the process of trying to conceive.

- **Engage in Relaxation Techniques:** Explore relaxation techniques such as meditation, yoga, or deep breathing to reduce stress and promote emotional well-being. These practices can help you calm your mind, relax your body, and find a sense of inner peace amidst the challenges of trying to conceive.
- **Pursue Hobbies and Interests:** Find joy and fulfillment by engaging in hobbies and interests

outside of the realm of trying to conceive. Whether it's painting, playing a musical instrument, or hiking in nature, pursuing activities that bring you happiness can provide a welcome distraction and a sense of fulfillment.

Additionally, it's important to prioritize self-care in other aspects of your life. This includes maintaining a healthy lifestyle through regular exercise, eating nutritious foods, and getting enough sleep. Taking care of your physical health can have a positive impact on your emotional well-being.

Remember, self-care is not selfish. It is a necessary part of the journey of trying to conceive. By prioritizing your own well-being, you are better equipped to navigate the emotional challenges that may arise along the way.

Engaging in Relaxation Techniques

Engaging in relaxation techniques can be a powerful tool for reducing stress and promoting emotional well-being during the journey of trying to conceive. One effective technique is meditation, which involves focusing the mind and achieving a state of deep relaxation. By setting aside a few minutes each day to meditate, couples can create a calm and peaceful environment that allows them to let go of stress and anxiety.

Another beneficial relaxation technique is practicing yoga. Yoga combines physical postures, breathing exercises, and meditation to improve flexibility, strength, and mental clarity. By incorporating yoga into their daily routine, couples can not only reduce stress but also enhance their overall well-being.

Deep breathing exercises are also a simple yet powerful relaxation technique. By taking slow, deep breaths and focusing on the breath entering and leaving the body, couples can activate the body's relaxation response, which helps to reduce stress and promote a sense of calm.

It's important for couples to explore different relaxation techniques and find what works best for them. Whether it's meditation, yoga, deep breathing, or a combination of these practices, engaging in relaxation techniques can provide a much-needed break from the emotional rollercoaster of trying to conceive and promote a sense of peace and well-being.

Pursuing Hobbies and Interests

Pursuing hobbies and interests outside of the realm of trying to conceive can bring joy and fulfillment to couples on their journey. It's important to remember that life is not solely defined by the quest for parenthood. Engaging in activities that bring happiness and fulfillment can help create a sense of balance and provide a much-needed distraction from the emotional rollercoaster.

One way to explore new hobbies is by creating a list of activities you've always wanted to try. Whether it's painting, photography, cooking, or learning a musical instrument, pursuing these interests can provide a sense of purpose and accomplishment. Consider taking a class or joining a club to connect with others who share your passion.

Additionally, spending time in nature can be incredibly therapeutic. Going for walks, hiking, or gardening can help reduce stress and promote a sense of calm. Being in nature allows you to disconnect from the pressures of trying to conceive and connect with the beauty of the world around you.

Another way to find joy and fulfillment is by giving back to the community. Volunteering for a cause you care about not only helps others but also provides a sense of fulfillment and purpose. It can be a rewarding experience to make a positive impact in the lives of others while navigating the challenges of trying to conceive.

Remember, pursuing hobbies and interests is not a distraction from the goal of becoming parents, but rather a way to nurture your own well-being and happiness. By finding joy and fulfillment outside of the realm of trying to conceive, you can create a more balanced and fulfilling life, regardless of the outcome of your journey.

Communicating with Your Partner

Nurturing open and honest communication with your partner is essential when navigating the emotional challenges of trying to conceive. The journey to parenthood can be filled with ups and downs, and having a strong foundation of communication can help you both navigate these challenges together.

One important aspect of communication is expressing your emotions and feelings. It's natural to experience a range of emotions throughout the process, from hope and excitement to frustration and disappointment. By openly expressing how you're feeling, you allow your partner to understand and support you better. This can help strengthen your bond and create a safe space for both of you to share your thoughts and concerns.

It's also important to listen actively to your partner. Give them the opportunity to express their emotions and concerns without judgment. Show empathy and validate their feelings, even if they differ from your own. This will foster a sense of understanding and create a supportive environment for both of you.

Creating regular opportunities for open and honest conversations is crucial. Set aside dedicated time to talk about your experiences, fears, and hopes regarding the journey to conception. This can be during a quiet evening at home or a date night out. By prioritizing these conversations, you show your commitment to working through the emotional challenges together.

Additionally, it can be helpful to establish shared goals and plans. Discuss your expectations, desires, and any potential changes or adjustments you may need to make along the way. This will help you both stay on the same page and make decisions together as a team.

Remember, open and honest communication is a two-way street. Be receptive to your partner's thoughts and feelings, and encourage them to do the same for you. By nurturing this type of communication, you can navigate the emotional rollercoaster of trying to conceive together, strengthening your relationship in the process.

Expressing Emotions

Expressing emotions is a crucial aspect of navigating the emotional rollercoaster of trying to conceive. It is important for partners to create a safe and supportive environment where they can openly express their emotions and feelings. By encouraging open communication, they can foster understanding and support for each other.

One way to encourage the expression of emotions is by setting aside dedicated time for honest conversations. This can be done through regular check-ins or designated "emotional sharing" sessions. During these times, partners can take turns expressing their thoughts, fears, hopes, and frustrations. Active listening and validation are key components of these conversations, as they help create a sense of empathy and understanding.

Creating a non-judgmental space is also essential. Both partners should feel comfortable sharing their emotions without fear of criticism or judgment. This can be achieved by practicing empathy and compassion towards each other's experiences. It is important to remember that everyone's emotions are valid and should be respected.

Additionally, using non-verbal forms of expression can also be helpful. Some individuals find it easier to express their emotions through writing, drawing, or other creative outlets. These activities can provide a sense of release and allow for deeper exploration of emotions.

By encouraging and embracing the open expression of emotions, partners can strengthen their bond and navigate the challenges of trying to conceive together. It allows them to gain a deeper understanding of each other's experiences and provides a foundation of support as they navigate the ups and downs of the journey.

Managing Differences in Coping

Managing Differences in Coping

When it comes to the emotional rollercoaster of trying to conceive, each partner may have their own unique way of coping. It's important to recognize and address these differences in order to find common ground and provide support for one another.

One partner may prefer to openly express their emotions and talk about their frustrations and disappointments, while the other may prefer to internalize their feelings and process them internally. This difference in coping mechanisms can sometimes lead to misunderstandings or feelings of disconnect between partners.

To navigate these differences, open and honest communication is key. Take the time to listen to each other's perspectives and validate each other's feelings. It's important to create a safe space where both partners feel comfortable expressing their emotions without judgment or criticism.

Additionally, finding common ground and compromise is essential. Explore activities or strategies that both partners can engage in together to support each other's emotional well-being. This could be as simple as going for walks together, practicing relaxation techniques, or engaging in a shared hobby or interest.

Remember, the journey of trying to conceive can be emotionally challenging for both partners, and it's important to be patient and understanding with each other. By addressing and managing differences in coping, you can strengthen your bond as a couple and navigate the emotional rollercoaster together.

Exploring the Decision to Stop Trying

Exploring the Decision to Stop Trying

Navigating the difficult decision of when to stop trying to conceive can be a challenging and emotional journey. For couples who have been trying to conceive for an extended period of time without success, the decision to stop can bring a mix of relief, sadness, and uncertainty. It is important for couples to give themselves permission to explore their feelings and come to a decision that feels right for them.

When faced with the decision to stop trying to conceive, couples may experience a range of emotions. There may be a sense of grief and loss for the dream of having a biological child. It can be difficult to let go of the hope and expectations that have been built up over time. It is important to acknowledge and process these emotions, allowing oneself to grieve and heal.

Communicating openly and honestly with one's partner is crucial during this time. It is important to have open discussions about the emotional toll that trying to conceive has taken and to explore the options and possibilities moving forward. Each partner may have different feelings and perspectives, and it is important to listen and validate each other's experiences.

Seeking support from loved ones, friends, or a therapist can also be beneficial during this time. Talking through one's feelings and concerns with a trusted confidant can provide valuable insight and perspective. Support groups for couples who have made the decision to stop trying to conceive can also be a source of comfort and understanding.

Ultimately, finding peace with the decision to stop trying to conceive is a personal journey. It may involve exploring other paths to fulfillment and happiness outside of parenthood. It may involve redefining what family means and embracing alternative paths such as adoption or assisted reproductive technologies. It is important to remember that there is no right or wrong decision, and each couple must do what feels right for them.

Grieving the Dream

Grieving the Dream

Deciding to stop trying to conceive can be an incredibly difficult and emotional decision. It means letting go of the dream of becoming parents and accepting that it may not happen biologically. This realization can bring about a range of complex emotions, including grief and loss.

Grief is a natural response to any kind of loss, and the loss of the dream of parenthood is no exception. It is important to acknowledge and process these emotions in order to heal and move forward. Grieving the dream involves allowing yourself to feel the sadness, disappointment, and even anger that may arise.

There is no right or wrong way to grieve, and everyone's experience is unique. Some individuals may find comfort in talking openly about their feelings, while others may prefer to process their emotions privately. It can be helpful to seek support from loved ones, friends, or a therapist who can provide a safe space to express and navigate these emotions.

During the grieving process, it is important to be gentle with yourself and give yourself permission to mourn the loss of the dream. This may involve taking time for self-care activities that bring you comfort and solace. Engaging in activities such as journaling, practicing mindfulness, or seeking solace in nature can help in the healing process.

It is also important to remember that grieving the dream does not mean giving up on happiness or fulfillment. It means redirecting your focus and exploring other paths to fulfillment and happiness outside of parenthood. This may involve pursuing new hobbies, interests, or goals that bring you joy and a sense of purpose.

Ultimately, grieving the dream is a deeply personal and individual process. It takes time, patience, and self-compassion. It is important to remember that it is okay to mourn the loss of the dream while also finding new ways to embrace and celebrate the life you have.

Exploring Other Paths to Fulfillment

When the decision to stop trying to conceive is made, it can be a challenging and emotional time for couples. However, it's important to remember that there are many other paths to fulfillment and happiness outside of parenthood. By considering and embracing these alternative paths, couples can find new sources of joy and purpose in their lives.

One option to explore is focusing on personal growth and self-discovery. This can involve pursuing new hobbies or interests that bring fulfillment and a sense of accomplishment. Whether it's learning a new skill, picking up a creative outlet like painting or writing, or getting involved in a cause or community organization, engaging in activities that bring joy and fulfillment can help fill the void left by the decision to stop trying to conceive.

Additionally, couples can consider expanding their family through adoption or fostering. This allows them to experience the joys of parenthood and make a positive impact in a child's life, even if it's not through biological means. Adoption and fostering can be incredibly rewarding experiences, providing a loving home to a child in need and creating a new chapter of love and growth for the couple.

Another alternative path to explore is focusing on building a strong and fulfilling relationship with your partner. Without the pressures and stresses of trying to conceive, couples can invest more time and energy into nurturing their bond. This can involve going on romantic dates, taking trips together, or even seeking couples therapy to strengthen communication and emotional connection. By prioritizing the relationship, couples can find fulfillment and happiness in the love they share.

Ultimately, the decision to stop trying to conceive opens up a world of possibilities for couples. It's important to remember that fulfillment and happiness can be found in many different ways, and parenthood is just one of them. By considering and embracing other paths, couples can find new sources of joy, purpose, and fulfillment in their lives.

Frequently Asked Questions

- **Q: How long does it typically take to conceive?**

  A: The time it takes to conceive can vary greatly from couple to couple. On average, it can take up to six months to a year of trying before successfully conceiving. However, it's important to remember that each person's fertility journey is unique.

- **Q: What are some common causes of infertility?**

  A: There are several factors that can contribute to infertility. Some common causes include hormonal imbalances, ovulation disorders, blocked fallopian tubes, low sperm count or quality, and age-related decline in fertility. It's best to consult with a healthcare professional for a thorough evaluation if you suspect infertility.

- **Q: How can I cope with the emotional toll of trying to conceive?**

  A: Coping with the emotional rollercoaster of trying to conceive can be challenging. It's important to find healthy coping mechanisms such as seeking support from loved ones, joining support groups, practicing self-care activities like yoga or meditation, and considering professional counseling or therapy when needed.

- **Q: When should I consider alternative paths to parenthood?**

  A: If conception proves difficult, it may be worth exploring alternative paths to parenthood such as adoption or assisted reproductive technologies. This decision is deeply personal and should be made after careful consideration and discussions with your partner and healthcare professionals.

- **Q: How can I manage jealousy and resentment towards others who achieve pregnancy?**

  A: It's natural to feel jealousy and resentment when others around you achieve pregnancy or parenthood. To manage these emotions, it can be helpful to limit exposure to triggers like social media, shift your perspective by focusing on personal growth and happiness, and seek support from your partner, friends, or support groups.

- **Q: How do I communicate with my partner about the emotional challenges?**

  A: Open and honest communication is key when navigating the emotional challenges of trying to conceive. Encourage each other to express emotions and feelings, and find common ground when coping strategies differ. Remember to support and comfort each other throughout the journey.

- **Q: How do I know when to stop trying to conceive?**

  A: Deciding when to stop trying to conceive is a deeply personal decision that varies for each individual or couple. It's important to consider factors such as physical and emotional well-being, financial implications, and alternative paths to fulfillment. Seek guidance from healthcare professionals and take time to reflect on what feels right for you.

Have Questions / Comments?

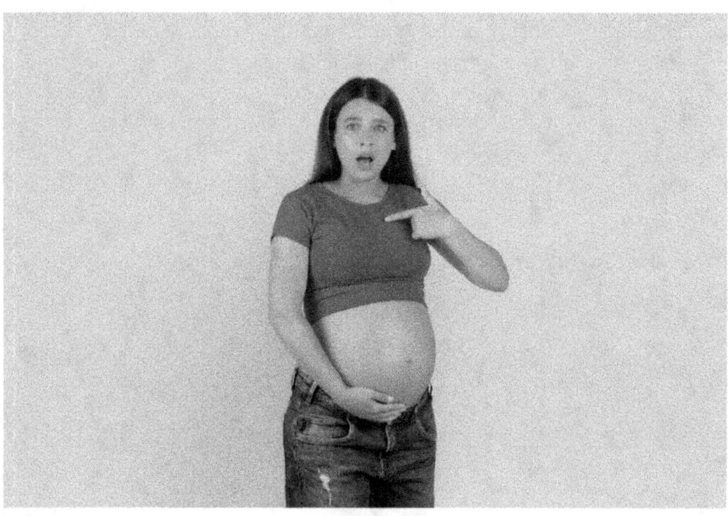

This book was designed to cover as much info as possible but I know I have probably missed something, or some new amazing discovery that has just come out.

If you notice something missing or have a question that I failed to answer, please get in touch and let me know. If I can, I will email you an answer and also update the book so others can also benefit from it.

Thanks For Being Awesome :)

Submit Your Questions / Comments At:

Get In Touch at Babydreamers.net

Get How To Be A Super Mom - 100% FREE

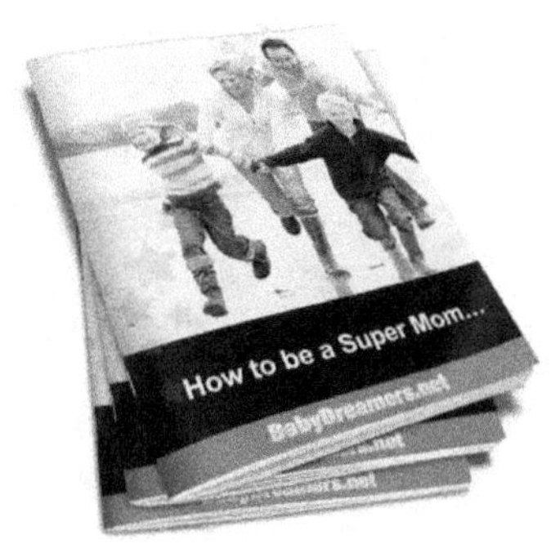

For being one of our amazing readers, we would love to offer you another book we have created, 100% free.

Being a mom is probably the most important job in the world – we've all heard that, and it's true. You're bringing up the next generation of wonderful, intelligent, loving, creative, responsible people.

We all want to be Super Mom and to be everything and do everything, but it this possible?

Being a Super Mom is possible, but you have to learn how to empower yourself to be the kind of Super Mom that you feel you need to be, keeping in mind that the title Super Mom doesn't mean the same thing to everyone.

<u>Get How to be a Super Mom For Free</u> at

BabyDreamers.net